T0224955

Cambridge Elements ☰

Elements in Emergency Neurosurgery
edited by
Nihal Gurusinghe
Lancashire Teaching Hospital NHS Trust
Peter Hutchinson
University of Cambridge, Society of British Neurological Surgeons and Royal College of Surgeons of England
Ioannis Fouyas
Royal College of Surgeons of Edinburgh
Naomi Slator
North Bristol NHS Trust
Ian Kamaly-Asl
Royal Manchester Children's Hospital
Peter Whitfield
University Hospitals Plymouth NHS Trust

ACUTE SPONTANEOUS POSTERIOR FOSSA HAEMORRHAGE

Lauren Harris
National Hospital for Neurology and Neurosurgery
Patrick Grover
National Hospital for Neurology and Neurosurgery

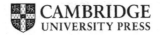
CAMBRIDGE
UNIVERSITY PRESS

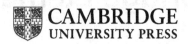

Shaftesbury Road, Cambridge CB2 8EA, United Kingdom

One Liberty Plaza, 20th Floor, New York, NY 10006, USA

477 Williamstown Road, Port Melbourne, VIC 3207, Australia

314–321, 3rd Floor, Plot 3, Splendor Forum, Jasola District Centre,
New Delhi – 110025, India

103 Penang Road, #05–06/07, Visioncrest Commercial, Singapore 238467

Cambridge University Press is part of Cambridge University Press & Assessment,
a department of the University of Cambridge.

We share the University's mission to contribute to society through the pursuit of
education, learning and research at the highest international levels of excellence.

www.cambridge.org
Information on this title: www.cambridge.org/9781009456487

DOI: 10.1017/9781009456456

First published 2024

A catalogue record for this publication is available from the British Library.

ISBN 978-1-009-45648-7 Hardback
ISBN 978-1-009-45650-0 Paperback
ISSN 2755-0656 (online)
ISSN 2755-0648 (print)

Acute Spontaneous Posterior Fossa Haemorrhage

Elements in Emergency Neurosurgery

DOI: 10.1017/9781009456456
First published online: February 2024

Lauren Harris
National Hospital for Neurology and Neurosurgery

Patrick Grover
National Hospital for Neurology and Neurosurgery

Author for correspondence: Lauren Harris, lauren.harris7@nhs.net

Abstract: Non-traumatic posterior fossa haemorrhage accounts for approximately 10% of all intracranial haematomas and 1.5% of all strokes. In the posterior fossa, a small amount of mass effect can have dramatic effects, due to its small volume. This can be due to immediate transmission of pressure to the brainstem, or via occlusion of the aqueduct of Sylvius or compression of the fourth ventricle, leading to acute obstructive hydrocephalus, with the risk of tonsillar herniation. Timely investigations and management are essential to maximise good outcomes. This Element offers a brief overview of posterior fossa haemorrhage. It looks at the anatomy, aetiology, management, and surgical options, with a review of the available evidence to guide practice.

Keywords: neurosurgery, posterior fossa, haemorrhage, decompression, surgery

ISBNs: 9781009456487 (HB), 9781009456500 (PB), 9781009456456 (OC)
ISSNs: 2755-0656 (online), 2755-0648 (print)

Contents

Anatomy

The posterior fossa is bounded by the posterior surface of the petrous temporal bone anteriorly, the occipital bone posteriorly, and laterally by the squamous and mastoid parts of the temporal bone (Figure 1). It is located between the foramen magnum inferiorly, and the tentorium cerebelli superiorly. It contains the cerebellum and the brainstem (Figure 2).

The posterior fossa is characterised by Rhoton's rule of three (2):

Brainstem: midbrain, pons, medulla
Cerebellar surfaces: petrosal, tentorial, suboccipital
Cerebellar peduncles: superior, middle, inferior
Fissures: cerebellomesencephalic, cerebellopontine, cerebellomedullary
Arteries: superior cerebellar artery (SCA), anterior inferior cerebellar artery
   (AICA), posterior inferior cerebellar artery (PICA)
Venous draining groups: petrosal, galenic, tentorial

Aetiology

The most likely aetiology for a spontaneous posterior fossa haematoma is underlying hypertension. This is seen predominantly in the middle-age or older population, from rupture of microaneurysms along penetrating small vessels. It often originates in the dentate nuclei or pons. In younger patients, an underlying vascular lesion needs to be ruled out. For a subacute history, a haemorrhagic tumour remains high in the differential. A more extensive list follows:

Primary

- Hypertensive
- Small vessel disease
- Amyloid – very rare in posterior fossa

Other

- Coagulopathy – Antiplatelets, anticoagulants, cirrhosis, thrombocytopenia
- Sympathomimetic drugs – cocaine, amphetamines

Vascular

- Aneurysmal – posterior circulation
- Cavernoma
- AVM
- AVF

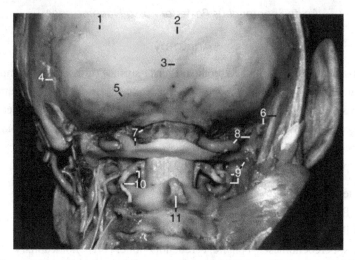

Figure 1 Posterior view of the posterior cranial fossa. All the suboccipital muscles have been removed. (a) Superior nuchal line; (b) external occipital protuberance; (c) external occipital crest; (d) occipitomastoid suture; (e) inferior nuchal line; (f) occipital artery and digastric muscle (posterior belly); (g) posterior arch of C1 and posterior meningeal artery piercing the posterior atlanto-occipital membrane; (h) vertebral artery and rectus capitis lateralis muscle; (i) transverse process of C1, anterior ramus of C2, and vertebral artery; (j) dorsal ganglion of C2 and posterior ramus of C2; (k) spinous process of C2 (3)

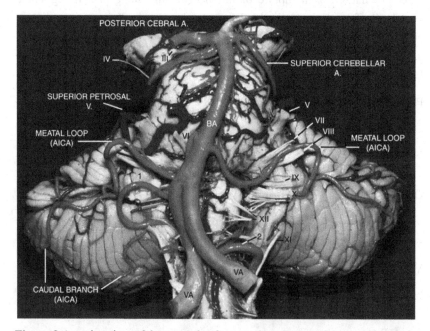

Figure 2 Anterior view of the posterior fossa to demonstrate the vascular supply and cranial nerves. (a) Flocculus; (b) posterior inferior cerebellar artery (PICA) (anterior medullary segment) (3).

- Haemorrhagic infarction – brainstem or cerebellar – embolic, thrombotic, vertebral artery dissection
- vasculitis

Trauma

- Subdural, extradural, or intra-axial – less than 3% of head injuries involve the posterior fossa (4)

Tumour

- Metastasis – melanoma, renal, lung, breast
- Haemangioblastoma – most common primary posterior fossa intra-axial tumour in adults
- Pilocytic astrocytoma
- Ependymoma
- Medulloblastoma
- Choroid plexus tumour – papilloma, carcinoma
- Brainstem glioma – rare in adults
- Dermoid/epidermoid
- Chordoma/chondrosarcoma

Infectious

- Abscess
- Septic emboli
- Encephalitis

Signs and Symptoms

The clinical presentation depends on the size of the haematoma (and associated oedema), what structures are involved, namely brainstem or cerebellar, and whether there is raised ICP from hydrocephalus. There is some overlap.

Raised ICP

- Headache – occipital
- Nausea/vomiting
- Neck pain or nuchal rigidity
- Papilloedema
- Gait disturbance
- Ataxia
- Vertigo

- Diplopia – VI nerve palsy
- Loss of consciousness with rapid deterioration into coma
- Tonsillar herniation 'coning' – where cerebellar tonsils herniate through the foramen magnum, compressing the medulla → Cushing response – sudden increase in BP, decrease in HR, and change in respiratory pattern → respiratory arrest

Cerebellar

- Ataxia
- Dysmetria
- Dysarthria
- Intention tremor
- Nystagmus
- Titubation

Brainstem

- Cranial nerve abnormalities – ophthalmoplegia, swallowing dysfunction
- Long-tract signs – tetraplegia, hemiplegia, extensor posturing
- Miosis
- Respiratory abnormalities – apneustic, cluster, or ataxic respirations
- Bradycardia, asystole

Management

As with all cases, management starts with an ABCDE assessment. Airway protection and intubation may be required for patients with a low Glasgow coma score (GCS). An assessment of neurology is made by GCS and pupil reaction. A rapid non-contrasted computed tomography (CT) head is required to identify the bleed. If there is a history of trauma, a full trauma CT including the cervical spine is warranted.

On CT, acute haemorrhage will appear hyperdense. It is important to appreciate if this is centred in the vermis, cerebellar hemispheres, or brainstem. Intraventricular or subarachnoid extension is common. The volume can be estimated using the ABC/2 formula. The degree of ventricle effacement, basal cistern effacement, brainstem compression, and hydrocephalus (alongside the patient's neurology) indicates the urgency of the situation, and is correlated with outcome.

Once a haemorrhagic cause is identified on imaging, it is important to reverse anticoagulation by usual methods (Table 1). Tranexamic acid – an antifibrinolytic that reversibly binds to plasminogen, preventing its conversion to plasmin, which degrades fibrin – can also be given.

Blood pressure control is mandatory, as these patients are often hypertensive. The National Institute for Health and Care Excellence (NICE) guidelines recommend a systolic of 140 mmHg or lower, whilst ensuring the BP does not drop more than 60 mmHg within one hour of starting treatment. This is not recommended if there is an underlying structural cause, if the GCS is <6, if surgery to evacuate the haematoma is imminent, or if there is a massive haematoma with likely poor prognosis (6). General neuroprotective measures are initiated, maintaining normal body temperature, normovolaemia, and normal glucose measurements (as hyperglycaemia has correlations with poor outcome) (7). The patient should be managed in a specialist Neuro ITU setting if appropriate.

Vascular imaging is recommended for anyone under the age of 45, or in 45–70 year olds without a history of hypertension (8). In reality, most patients have vascular imaging, usually in the form of a CT angiogram (CTA), as it is fast, non-invasive, accessible, and has a 96.6% sensitivity, and diagnostic accuracy of 96.9% (9). MR angiogram (MRA) is an alternative, often in a delayed setting following the resolution of the haematoma. Digital subtraction angiogram (DSA) is the gold standard, although there may not be time in

Table 1 Common anticoagulants and antiplatelets, their mechanism of action, and reversal agents. *Potential direct oral anticoagulant (DOAC) reversal agent under review (5).

Anticoagulant	Mechanism	Reversal agents
Warfarin	Vitamin K antagonist	Vitamin K, prothrombin complex concentrate (PCC), fresh frozen plasma
Heparin	Indirect thrombin inhibitor	Protamine
Dabigatran	Direct thrombin inhibitor	Idarucizumab, ciraparantag*
Apixaban/edoxaban/ rivaroxaban	Direct Xa inhibitor	Andexanet alfa, PCC, recombinant factor Xa, ciraparantag
Antiplatelet		
Aspirin	Cyclooxygenase inhibitor	Irreversible Platelets, desmopressin
Clopidogrel	ADP inhibitor (P2Y12) receptor	Irreversible Platelets

the emergency setting. It is performed in a stable patient, if the CTA suggests a vascular malformation.

If there is suspicion of an underlying lesion, and the patient is stable, an MRI head with and without contrast with stealth sequences can be done. A CT chest abdomen pelvis, and a multidisciplinary team (MDT) discussion with the oncologists is recommended to plan management, if time allows. There is no routine role for steroids in posterior fossa haematomas, unless there is a haemorrhagic tumour with surrounding oedema.

Indications for Surgery

1. Haematoma > 3 cm/15 mls if symptomatic or neurological dysfunction
2. Neurological deterioration related to the lesion
3. Mass effect on CT – distortion, dislocation, or obliteration of the 4th ventricle, compression or loss of visualisation of basal cisterns, obstructive hydrocephalus (10).

An emergency surgical decompression and evacuation is required, as the patient is at risk of rapid deterioration. This means any patient who is maintaining a good GCS but at risk of deterioration (e.g. headache only, drowsy, with a large clot) should be blue light transferred to a neurosurgical unit, ideally intensive care, for close observation, so that intervention can proceed on immediate deterioration.

A conservative approach is appropriate for patients with small clots <3 cm and good neurological function, with close neuro observation and serial imaging.

A harder clinical decision is when not to operate. Patients with a poor baseline, with many co-morbidities, are unlikely to benefit from a high-risk surgical intervention. If the presenting scan shows brainstem involvement, in the form of a brainstem haematoma, this implies irreversible damage, and surgery may not improve the outcome. These patients are usually managed conservatively. Patients with small bleeds, either hypertensive or from a small cavernoma, may make a reasonable recovery, and can be managed by the stroke team. If the brainstem haematoma is extensive, best supportive care, family discussion, brainstem testing, and early discussion with the organ donation team are appropriate. This can often be difficult in young patients with no previous past medical history. Brainstem haemorrhage must be differentiated from brainstem compression from adjacent mass effect/haematoma, which may improve with a decompression, if performed in a timely fashion.

Surgery

Posterior Fossa Craniectomy

Anaesthetic considerations include adequate anaesthesia, analgesia, mainten-ance of cerebral perfusion pressure (CPP), haemodynamic stability, and avoid-ance of cough. Brainstem manipulation may cause dysrhythmias (both bradycardias and tachycardias). Stimulation of trigemino-cardiac reflex can cause hypertension and bradycardia.

The patient is usually positioned prone, in the concorde position for midline lesions, on a Montreal mattress or equivalent. For hemispheric lesions, a lateral oblique (park bench) position can also be used. The patient's head is usually pinned with the Mayfield clamp with a single pin on the side of the lesion.

The incision is usually midline, starting at the C2 spinous process proceeding superiorly to the external occipital protuberance (inion). This should be extended at least 6 cm superiorly if a Frazier burr hole is to be done. A paramedian or hockey stick incision can be used for a hemispheric lesion.

The muscles and fascia are incised in the avascular midline, usually with monopolar, with a 'T' at the top, leaving a cuff of tissue above the superior nuchal line to help water tight closure. The muscles include the sternocleido-mastoid, trapezius, splenius capitis, semi spinalis, and the suboccipital muscles (rectus capitis posterior major, rectus capitis posterior minor, superior oblique capitis, and inferior oblique capitis). If a paramedian approach is required, then the muscles will be split accordingly.

A large midline suboccipital craniectomy is usually indicated, with removal of the bone, to accommodate post-operative swelling. For tumour resections, a craniotomy can be performed, depending on the clinical situation and anticipated swelling. The craniectomy margins are:

Superiorly: transverse sinus

> Inferior margin of the transverse sinus is in line with the zygoma and external acoustic meatus, two finger breaths above the mastoid notch – just above the superior nuchal line.

Inferiorly: foramen magnum
Laterally: sigmoid sinus

> Mastoid/digastric groove
> Must pack mastoid air cells with bone wax or muscle if entered to prevent CSF leak

In some situations (if tonsillar herniation is evident), removal of the posterior arch of C1 is also indicated, with care regarding the vertebral arteries on the superior aspect of C1.

A Y-shaped durotomy is often used, with additional releasing incisions if required. At this point, clot evacuation occurs, usually using suction and bipolar. For a haemorrhagic infarction resection of the damaged cerebellar tissue may be appropriate. Care should be taken if there is an underlying vascular lesion, and a neurovascular consultant should be present for the resection.

Haemostasis is vital. The small cavity of the posterior fossa can have devastating consequences if there is a post-operative haematoma. Special care needs to be taken for any coagulopathic patient. Numerous agents can be employed to help haemostasis, and the anaesthetist should slowly elevate the BP to test prior to closure. The dura is left open to allow for brain expansion, and the decision to use a dural graft or tissue glue is surgeon specific. A multi-layer meticulous muscle closure is required to reduce the risk of CSF leak.

External Ventricular Drain – Frazier Burr Hole

Hydrocephalus is frequently a component of posterior fossa haematomas, both obstructive hydrocephalus preoperatively and communicating hydrocephalus post-operatively, often if there's a heavy blood load. It is often recommended to do a prophylactic external ventricular drain (EVD) in addition to the suboccipital decompression and evacuation. This can be done through a standard frontal Kocher's burr hole with the patient supine (on the patient bed or operating table depending on urgency) prior to flipping the patient prone. Another faster, more convenient option, is an occipital Frazier burr hole.

Location: 3–4 cm from midline, 6–7 cm above inion in adults (2–3 cm above transverse sinus or 3–4 cm above inion in paediatrics).

This is performed when the patient is positioned prone. It is also used in an elective setting, for example for tumours, to mitigate post-operative swelling, or hydrocephalus. Neuronavigation can be used. It is often performed as the first step in the operation, prior to the suboccipital decompression.

Often CSF is drained only after the dura is opened. This theoretically avoids upwards herniation where the cerebellar vermis ascends above the tentorium, compressing the midbrain and superior cerebellar arteries, to help equalise the supra- and infratentorial pressure. Another option is to open the drain immediately at a high pressure, with cautious drainage of CSF.

Post-operatively, the drain is usually set at 10–15cmH$_2$O for 48–72 hours, and progressively raised depending on aetiology and neurology.

Post-operative management

- May need intubation, ventilation, and sedation on a Neuro ITU
- Avoid hypertension
- Close wound review
- Close neuro observation
- General neuroprotective measures
- Management of EVD

Specific post-operative complications

- Local pain as no bone flap
- Syndrome of the trephine
- CSF leak → meningitis
- Hydrocephalus
- Pseudomeningocele
- Swallowing difficulties – speech and language therapy (SALT) involvement
- Aspiration risk
- Vocal cord dysfunction

The Evidence

Unlike supratentorial strokes/haemorrhage, there have been no large randomised controlled trials (RCTs) for infratentorial decompression and clot evacuation. For cerebellar haematomas, outcome is related to neurological status. In a retrospective study of 81 patients, 95% had a favourable outcome (Glasgow outcome score (GOS) 4 or 5) if admission GCS was ≥ 8, versus 81% had a poor outcome (GOS 1–3) if GCS was <8 (11). Brainstem involvement is universally associated with poor outcome (12).

Treatment recommendations are based on meta-analysis of observational cohort studies, with associated risks of bias, and heterogeneity between studies (13). There is a general consensus that symptomatic cerebellar haematomas larger than 3 cm should be evacuated (14). Indications for decompressive surgery include neurological deterioration, brainstem compression, and hydrocephalus (10,15,16).

The degree of ventricular effacement is important and can be classified as grade I (normal), grade II (compressed), or grade III (completely effaced) (17). The degree of fourth ventricle compression is correlated with the size and volume of the haematoma, and the presenting GCS (17). If the patient has a good GCS, large haematomas can be successfully managed conservatively, as long as the fourth ventricle is not completely effaced (17). This study recommends evacuation in conscious patients if the ventricles are completely effaced, before deterioration (17).

A meta-analysis of 578 patients showed that surgical haematoma evacuation was associated with better survival at 3 and 12 months, but not significantly associated with better outcome at three months, versus conservative management (18). Mortality benefit occurred for patients with haematomas >15 ml, whilst those <12 ml had a lower likelihood of good surgical outcome (18). One retrospective study of 85 patients demonstrated improved mortality and functional outcomes for decompression and evacuation, versus evacuation alone (19). The perceived lack of equipoise regarding the life-saving benefit of surgery for cerebellar haematomas most likely means that a randomised clinical trial will not occur. Whether surgery improves functional outcome remains uncertain.

The 2022 American Heart Association/American Stroke Association guidelines recommend surgery (8):

> *'For patients with cerebellar ICH who are deteriorating neurologically, have brainstem compression and/or hydrocephalus from ventricular obstruction, or have cerebellar ICH volume ≥15 ml, immediate surgical removal of the haemorrhage with or without EVD is recommended in preference to medical management alone to reduce mortality.'*

The European stroke organisation guidelines conclude (20):

> *'There is insufficient evidence from RCTs to make strong recommendations about how, when, and for whom to perform surgical evacuation in adults with infratentorial ICH.'*

There is a general consensus that controlling ICP with an EVD alone is insufficient, potentially harmful, and not recommended (3). In one retrospective study of 104 patients, EVD alone had a significantly higher mortality versus decompression (47.8% v 17.4%, p = 0.008) or conservative management (45.7%) (21). The incidence of upward herniation after EVD insertion for posterior fossa lesions is unclear, but in the range of 3–8% (22–24).

There is no adequately powered study comparing different surgical approaches. One small RCT compared a paramedian suboccipital minicraniectomy with a large suboccipital craniectomy. It found no difference in overall outcome between the two groups, with fewer complications (less blood transfusions, shorter operation, less corticospinal fluid (CSF) leak) in the minicraniectomy group (25). Small retrospective studies have compared endoscopic or stereotactic aspiration with standard suboccipital decompression, with variable results (26–28). This is likely to be the focus of future work.

For pontine haemorrhage, a systematic review of 1,437 patients revealed an early mortality of 48.1%, with admission GCS and size predicting worse outcomes (29). Age, localisation, and intraventricular extension did not consistently predict prognosis (29). For acute hydrocephalus associated with pontine haemorrhage, no improvement in outcome has been found in patients treated with an EVD (30,31). The efficacy of surgery for pontine haematomas is inconclusive, with conflicting evidence from small studies in China, Japan, and South Korea (32–34). The largest study of 281 patients suggests surgical treatment is associated with a lower 30-day mortality, but no better 90-day functional recovery (31). There is currently a multi-centre, randomised, controlled, open-label trial (STIPE) taking place in China to compare primary pontine haematoma evacuation with medical management (35).

For cerebellar infarction, a 2018 systematic review of 283 patients showed poor outcomes after suboccipital decompressive craniectomy, with a 28% moderate to severe disability, and a 20% mortality (36). Mortality was lower with a mean age of less than 60, higher preoperative GCS, decompression within 48 hours of the ictus, concomitant EVD insertion, and debridement of the infarction (36). The data is mostly from small retrospective studies, with heterogeneity between studies. A retrospective case controlled study showed improved clinical outcomes (modified Rankin scale score 0–2 at 12 months, odds ratio 4.8, $p = 0.009$) in patients who underwent a suboccipital decompression (n = 28) versus conservative management (n = 56) for cerebellar infarction, in the absence of brainstem infarction (37).

Typical Clinical Scenarios

Hypertensive Bleed

A 59-year-old male presented with a sudden onset headache and collapsed 15 minutes later at home. He had no known past medical history. With the paramedic crew he had a GCS of 10 (E3V2M5) but dropped to GCS 3 on arrival at his local hospital. His pupils were 2 mm and sluggish. His systolic blood pressure was 215. He was intubated and ventilated. A CT head (Figure 3) showed acute blood within the cerebellar vermis, with extension into the ventricles, and the subarachnoid space. There was moderate tri-ventricular hydrocephalus and crowding of the foramen magnum. A CT angiogram showed a dilated vein entering the centre of the clot but no visible vascular malformation.

He was transferred as an emergency straight to theatre, and given 200 mls of 20% mannitol on route. He underwent a right frontal EVD, followed by a decompressive craniectomy and clot evacuation. Post-operatively he was managed in Neuro ITU. He had a post-operative DSA that was negative.

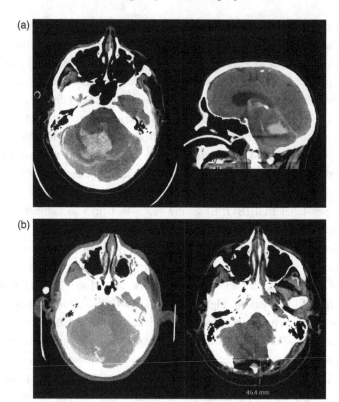

Figure 3 Hypertensive posterior fossa haematoma. (a) Axial CT showing diffuse posterior fossa haemorrhage with extension into the fourth ventricle. (b) Sagittal CT showing compression of the fourth ventricle with early hydrocephalus. (c) Axial CTA demonstrating a suspicious vascular structure of unknown significance. (d) Post-operative axial CT showing adequate decompression of the posterior fossa with clot evacuation.

One year post-operatively his recovery is ongoing. His language and memory are intact. He is PEG fed, and wheelchair bound, but can transfer.

Tumour

A 57-year-old male presented to the emergency department with a fall. He has had multiple falls over the last few weeks, and had become increasingly unsteady on his feet, requiring the use of a stick and assistance from his wife. Over the last week he has also been complaining of headache, with one episode of vomiting. He was on apixaban for atrial fibrillation, which was stopped on admission.

A trauma CT head (Figure 4) revealed a haemorrhagic lesion within the posterior fossa, to the right of the midline, with mixed density. There was surrounding

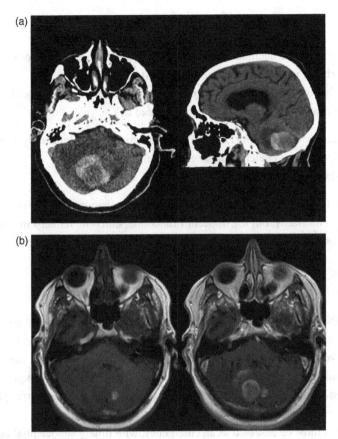

Figure 4 Posterior fossa haemorrhagic metastasis. (a) Axial CT demonstrating mixed density blood with surrounding oedema. (b) sagittal CT showing compression of the fourth ventricle. (c) Axial non-contrasted MRI head showing haemorrhagic lesion with surrounding oedema. (d) axial contrasted MRI showing some enhancement.

vasogenic oedema and associated mass effect with effacement of the fourth ventricle. An MRI head with and without contrast demonstrated the solitary lesion further, centred in the vermis, with extension into the right cerebellar hemisphere, measuring 4.5 cm in largest diameter. CT chest abdomen pelvis showed a 17-mm lung nodule, a 23-mm pretracheal lymph node, and a 10-mm focal hepatic lesion.

He underwent an image guided right posterior fossa craniotomy for tumour. A prophylactic Frazier burr hole EVD was performed, with the drain left clamped. It was removed on day 3, and he was discharged following therapy input, with improved gait. Histology revealed an underlying melanoma metastasis, which is being treated.

Important Points

1. Posterior fossa haematomas are usually hypertensive in aetiology, but an underlying vascular cause or tumour must be considered.
2. Timely intervention in the form of a suboccipital decompression and haematoma evacuation +/– EVD is recommended if:

   a. Haematoma > 3 cm/15 mls if symptomatic or neurological dysfunction
   b. Neurological deterioration related to the lesion
   c. Mass effect on CT

3. No RCTs are available to guide treatment decisions. Surgery appears to reduce mortality, but the impact of functional outcome remains uncertain.
4. Brainstem involvement is a poor prognostic feature, and many of these patients are managed conservatively with best supportive care.

Conclusion

Posterior fossa haematomas are often hypertensive in aetiology, but an underlying vascular cause or tumour must be considered. The posterior fossa has a small volume, so a bleed can be devastating. This can be due to immediate transmission of pressure to the brainstem, or via occlusion of the aqueduct or compression of the fourth ventricle, leading to acute obstructive hydrocephalus, with the risk of tonsillar herniation.

Patients must be assessed as an emergency, with timely suboccipital decompression and evacuation +/– EVD for suitable patients. No RCTs are available to guide treatment decisions. Surgery appears to reduce mortality, but the impact of functional outcome remains uncertain.

References

1. Hemphill JC, Amin-Hanjani S. Cerebellar Intracerebral Hemorrhage: Time for Evidence-Based Treatment. JAMA [Internet]. 8 October 2019 [cited 13 March 2023];322(14):1355–6. US, New York. https://jamanetwork.com/journals/jama/fullarticle/2752450.

2. Rhoton AL, Jr. Rhoton's Cranial Anatomy and Surgical Approaches [Internet]. 2007 [cited 13 March 2023]. p. 746. http://books.google.com/books?id=ERKbHwAACAAJ&pgis=1.

3. Winn R. Youmans and Winn Neurological Surgery [Internet]. 8th ed. Elsevier; 2022 [cited 13 March 2023]. https://bookshelf.health.elsevier.com/reader/books/9780323675000/epubcfi/6/1124[%3Bvnd.vst.idref%3DB9780323661928004067]!/4/2[c0406]/8/4/6/254[bib126]/6/1:93[ent%2Cof].

4. Greenberg MS. Greenberg's Handbook of Neurosurgery – 9th Edition: Handbook of Neurosurgery. Thieme Medical Publisher; 2020.

5. Ansell J, Laulicht BE, Bakhru SH, et al. Ciraparantag, an Anticoagulant Reversal Drug: Mechanism of Action, Pharmacokinetics, and Reversal of Anticoagulants. Blood [Internet]. 7 January 2021 [cited 2 April 2023];137(1):115–25. https://pubmed.ncbi.nlm.nih.gov/33205809/.

6. NICE. Recommendations | Stroke and Transient Ischaemic Attack in over 16s: Diagnosis and Initial Management | Guidance | NICE. 2022.

7. Wu YT, Li TY, Lu SC, et al. Hyperglycemia as a Predictor of Poor Outcome at Discharge in Patients with Acute Spontaneous Cerebellar Hemorrhage. Cerebellum [Internet]. June 2012 [cited 13 March 2023];11(2):543–8. https://pubmed.ncbi.nlm.nih.gov/21975857/.

8. Greenberg SM, Ziai WC, Cordonnier C, et al. 2022 Guideline for the Management of Patients with Spontaneous Intracerebral Hemorrhage: A Guideline from the American Heart Association/American Stroke Association. Stroke [Internet]. 1 July 2022 [cited 13 March 2023];53(7):E282–361. www.ahajournals.org/doi/abs/10.1161/STR.0000000000000407.

9. Vignesh S, Prasad SN, Singh V, et al. Angiographic Analysis on Posterior Fossa Hemorrhages and Vascular Malformations beyond Aneurysms by CT Angiography and Digital Subtraction Angiography. Egypt J Neurosurg 2022 371 [Internet]. 18 April 2022 [cited 14 March 2023];37(1):1–9. https://ejns.springeropen.com/articles/10.1186/s41984-022-00152-2.

10. Bullock MR, Chesnut R, Ghajar J et al. Surgical Management of Posterior Fossa Mass Lesions. Neurosurgery [Internet]. 2006 [cited 13 March 2023];58: S47–55. www.neurosurgery-online.com.

11. D'Avella D, Servadei F, Scerrati M, et al. Traumatic Intracerebellar Hemorrhage: Clinicoradiological Analysis of 81 Patients. Neurosurgery [Internet]. January 2002 [cited 13 March 2023];50(1):16–25. https:// pubmed.ncbi.nlm.nih.gov/11844230/.

12. Yanaka K, Meguro K, Fujita K, Narushima K, Nose T. Postoperative Brainstem High Intensity Is Correlated with Poor Outcomes for Patients with Spontaneous Cerebellar Hemorrhage. Neurosurgery [Internet]. 1999 [cited 13 March 2023];45(6):1323–8. https://pubmed.ncbi.nlm.nih.gov/ 10598699/.

13. Singh SD, Brouwers HB, Senff JR, et al. Haematoma Evacuation in Cerebellar Intracerebral Haemorrhage: Systematic Review. J Neurol Neurosurg Psychiatry [Internet]. 1 January 2020 [cited 13 March 2023];91(1):82–7. https://pubmed.ncbi.nlm.nih.gov/31848229/.

14. Koziarski A, Frankiewicz E. Medical and Surgical Treatment of Intracerebellar Haematomas. Acta Neurochir (Wien) [Internet]. March 1991 [cited 13 March 2023];110(1–2):24–8. https://pubmed.ncbi.nlm.nih.gov/ 1882714/.

15. Dammann P, Asgari S, Bassiouni H, et al. Spontaneous Cerebellar Hemorrhage–Experience with 57 Surgically Treated Patients and Review of the Literature. *Neurosurg Rev [Internet]*. January 2011 [cited 13 March 2023];34(1):77–86. https://pubmed.ncbi.nlm.nih.gov/20697766/.

16. Da Pian R, Bazzan A, Pasqualin A. Surgical Versus Medical Treatment of Spontaneous Posterior Fossa Haematomas: A Cooperative Study on 205 Cases. Neurol Res [Internet]. 1984 [cited 13 March 2023];6(3):145–51 https://pubmed.ncbi.nlm.nih.gov/6151139/.

17. Kirollos RW, Tyagi AK, Ross SA, et al. Management of Spontaneous Cerebellar Hematomas: A Prospective Treatment Protocol. Neurosurgery [Internet]. 2001 [cited 2023 Mar 13];49(6):1378–87. https://pubmed.ncbi .nlm.nih.gov/11846937/.

18. Kuramatsu JB, Biffi A, Gerner ST, et al. Association of Surgical Hematoma Evacuation vs Conservative Treatment with Functional Outcome in Patients with Cerebellar Intracerebral Hemorrhage. JAMA [Internet]. 8 October 2019 [cited 13 March 2023];322(14):1392–403. https://pubmed .ncbi.nlm.nih.gov/31593272/.

19. Hackenberg KAM, Unterberg AW, Jung CS, et al. Does Suboccipital Decompression and Evacuation of Intraparenchymal Hematoma Improve Neurological Outcome in Patients with Spontaneous Cerebellar

Hemorrhage? Clin Neurol Neurosurg [Internet]. 1 April 2017 [cited 14 March 2023];155:22–9. https://pubmed.ncbi.nlm.nih.gov/28226284/.

20. Steiner T, Al-Shahi Salman R, Beer R, et al. European Stroke Organisation (ESO) Guidelines for the Management of Spontaneous Intracerebral Hemorrhage. Int J Stroke [Internet]. 1 October 2014 [cited 13 March 2023];9(7):840–55. https://journals.sagepub.com/doi/10.1111/ijs.12309? icid=int.sj-full-text.similar-articles.3.

21. Luney MS, English SW, Longworth A, et al. Acute Posterior Cranial Fossa Hemorrhage – Is Surgical Decompression Better than Expectant Medical Management? Neurocrit Care [Internet]. 1 December 2016 [cited 14 March 2023];25(3):365. /pmc/articles/PMC5138260/.

22. Braksick SA, Himes BT, Snyder K, et al Ventriculostomy and Risk of Upward Herniation in Patients with Obstructive Hydrocephalus from Posterior Fossa Mass Lesions. Neurocrit Care [Internet]. 1 June 2018 [cited 14 March 2023];28(3):338–43. https://pubmed.ncbi.nlm.nih.gov/ 29305758/.

23. Raimondi AJ, Tomita T. Hydrocephalus and Infratentorial Tumors: Incidence, Clinical Picture, and Treatment. J Neurosurg [Internet]. 1 August 1981 [cited 14 March 2023];55(2):174–82. https://thejns.org/ view/journals/j-neurosurg/55/2/article-p174.xml.

24. Moscardini-Martelli J, Ponce-Gomez JA, Alcocer-Barradas V, et al. Upward Transtentorial Herniation: A New Role for Endoscopic Third Ventriculostomy. Surg Neurol Int [Internet]. 2021 [cited 14 March 2023];12(334). /pmc/articles/ PMC8326076/.

25. Tamaki T, Kitamura T, Node Y, Teramoto A. Paramedian Suboccipital Mini-Craniectomy for Evacuation of Spontaneous Cerebellar Hemorrhage. Neurol Med Chir (Tokyo) [Internet]. November 2004 [cited 13 March 2023]; 44(11):578–82. https://pubmed.ncbi.nlm.nih.gov/15686176/.

26. Tokimura H, Tajitsu K, Taniguchi A, et al. Efficacy and Safety of Key Hole Craniotomy for the Evacuation of Spontaneous Cerebellar Hemorrhage. *Neurol Med Chir (Tokyo) [Internet]*. 1 January 2010 [cited 13 March 2023]; 50(5):367–72. https://europepmc.org/article/MED/20505290.

27. Kellner CP, Moore F, Arginteanu MS, et al. Minimally Invasive Evacuation of Spontaneous Cerebellar Intracerebral Hemorrhage. World Neurosurg [Internet]. 3 October 2018 [cited 13 March 2023];122:e1–9. https://eur opepmc.org/article/MED/30292039.

28. Khattar NK, Fortuny EM, Wessell AP, et al. Minimally Invasive Surgery for Spontaneous Cerebellar Hemorrhage: A Multicenter Study. World Neurosurg [Internet]. 1 September 2019 [cited 13 March 2023];129:e35–9. https://pubmed.ncbi.nlm.nih.gov/31042595/.

29. Behrouz R. Prognostic Factors in Pontine Haemorrhage: A Systematic Review. Eur stroke J [Internet]. 1 June 2018 [cited 14 March 2023]; 3(2):101–9. https://pubmed.ncbi.nlm.nih.gov/31008342/.

30. Murata Y, Yamaguchi S, Kajikawa H, et al. Relationship between the Clinical Manifestations, Computed Tomographic Findings and the Outcome in 80 Patients with Primary Pontine Hemorrhage. J Neurol Sci [Internet]. 15 August 1999 [cited 14 March 2023];167(2):107–11. www.jns-journal.com/article/S0022510X99001501/fulltext.

31. Jang JH, Song YG, Kim YZ. Predictors of 30-Day Mortality and 90-Day Functional Recovery after Primary Pontine Hemorrhage. J Korean Med Sci [Internet]. January 2011 [cited 14 March 2023];26(1):100. /pmc/articles/PMC3012832.

32. Chen P, Yao H, Tang X, et al. Management of Primary Brainstem Hemorrhage: A Review of Outcome Prediction, Surgical Treatment, and Animal Model. Dis Markers [Internet]. 2022 [cited 14 March 2023];2022. /pmc/articles/PMC9296309/.

33. Ichimura S, Bertalanffy H, Nakaya M, et al. Surgical Treatment for Primary Brainstem Hemorrhage to Improve Postoperative Functional Outcomes. World Neurosurg. 1 December 2018;120:e1289–94.

34. Chen D, Tang Y, Nie H, et al. Primary Brainstem Hemorrhage: A Review of Prognostic Factors and Surgical Management. *Front Neurol [Internet]*. 10 September 2021 [cited 14 March 2023]; 12. https://pubmed.ncbi.nlm.nih.gov/34566872/.

35. He Q, Wang J, Ma L, Li H, Tao C, You C. Safety of Surgical Treatment in Severe Primary Pontine Haemorrhage Evacuation (STIPE): Study Protocol for a Multi-Centre, Randomised, Controlled, Open-Label Trial. BMJ Open [Internet]. 23 August 2022 [cited 14 March 2023];12(8). https://pubmed.ncbi.nlm.nih.gov/35998952/.

36. Ayling OGS, Alotaibi NM, Wang JZ, et al. Suboccipital Decompressive Craniectomy for Cerebellar Infarction: A Systematic Review and Meta-Analysis. World Neurosurg [Internet]. 1 February 2018 [cited 13 March 2023]; 110:450–459.e5. https://pubmed.ncbi.nlm.nih.gov/29104155/.

37. Kim MJ, Park SK, Song J, et al. Preventive Suboccipital Decompressive Craniectomy for Cerebellar Infarction: A Retrospective-Matched Case-Control Study. Stroke [Internet]. 1 October 2016 [cited 13 March 2023]; 47(10):2565–73. https://pubmed.ncbi.nlm.nih.gov/27608818/.

Emergency Neurosurgery

Nihal Gurusinghe

Lancashire Teaching Hospital NHS Trust

Professor Nihal Gurusinghe is a Consultant Neurosurgeon at the Lancashire Teaching Hospitals NHS Trust. He is on the Executive Council of the Society of British Neurological Surgeons as the Lead for NICE (National Institute for Health and Care Excellence) guidelines relating to neurosurgical practice. He is also an examiner for the UK and International FRCS examinations in Neurosurgery.

Peter Hutchinson

University of Cambridge, Society of British Neurological Surgeons and Royal College of Surgeons of England

Peter Hutchinson (BSc MBBS FFSEM FRCS(SN) PhD FMedSci) is Professor of Neurosurgery and Head of the Division of Academic Neurosurgery at the University of Cambridge, and Honorary Consultant Neurosurgeon at Addenbrooke's Hospital. He is Director of Clinical Research at the Royal College of Surgeons of England and Meetings Secretary of the Society of British Neurological Surgeons.

Ioannis Fouyas

Royal College of Surgeons of Edinburgh

Ioannis Fouyas is a Consultant Neurosurgeon in Edinburgh. His clinical interests focus on the treatment of complex cerebrovascular and skull base pathologies. His academic endeavours concentrate in the field of cerebrovascular pathophysiology. His passion is technical surgical training, fulfilled in collaboration with the Royal College of Surgeons of Edinburgh. Finally, he pursues Undergraduate Neuroscience teaching, with a particular focus on functional Neuroanatomy.

Naomi Slator

North Bristol NHS Trust

Naomi Slator FRCS (SN) is a Consultant Spinal Neurosurgeon based at North Bristol NHS Trust. She has a specialist interest in Complex Spine alongside Cranial and Spinal Trauma. She completed her neurosurgical training in Birmingham and a six-month Fellowship in CSF and Trauma (2019). She then went on to complete her Spinal Fellowship in Leeds (2020) before moving to the southwest to take up her consultant post.

Ian Kamaly-Asl

Royal Manchester Children's Hospital

Ian Kamaly-Asl is a full-time paediatric neurosurgeon and Honorary Chair at Royal Manchester Children's Hospital. He trained in North Western Deanery with fellowships at Boston Children's Hospital and Sick Kids in Toronto. Ian is a member of council of The Royal College of Surgeons of England and the SBNS where he is lead for mentoring and tackling oppressive behaviours.

Peter Whitfield

University Hospitals Plymouth NHS Trust

Professor Peter Whitfield is a Consultant Neurosurgeon at the South West Neurosurgical Centre, University Hospitals Plymouth NHS Trust. His clinical interests include vascular neurosurgery, neuro oncology, and trauma. He has held many roles in postgraduate neurosurgical education and is President of the Society of British Neurological Surgeons. Peter has published widely and is passionate about education, training, and the promotion of clinical research.

About the Series

Elements in Emergency Neurosurgery is intended for trainees and practitioners in Neurosurgery and Emergency Medicine as well as allied specialties all over the world. Authored by international experts, this series provides core knowledge, common clinical pathways, and recommendations on the management of acute conditions of the brain and spine.

Cambridge Elements ≡

Emergency Neurosurgery

Elements in the Series

A full series listing is available at: www.cambridge.org/EEMN